Stomach Ulcer Diet Cookbook

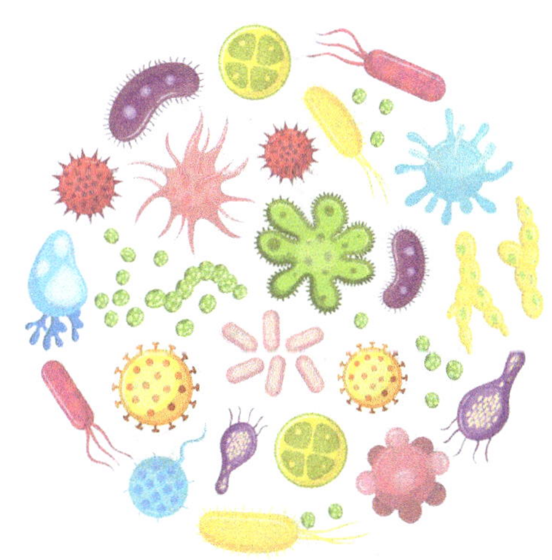

Smoothies, Tea, Anti-inflammatory Drinks and Probiotics for Managing Gut Health

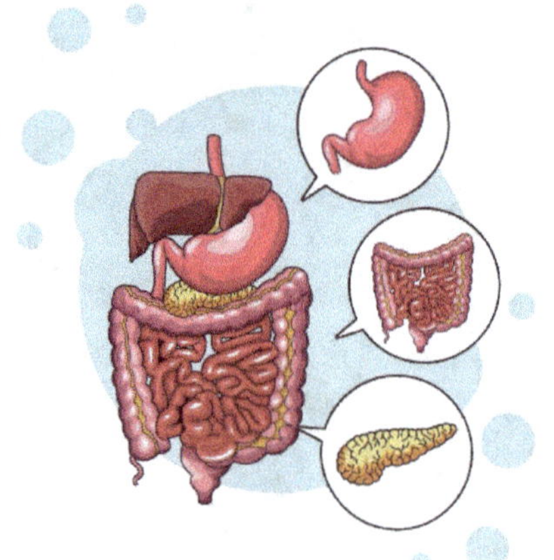

ISBN: 9798392005406

This book is dedicated to those stomach ulcer sufferers who are looking for a dietary strategy to control their illness. May this cookbook serve as a source of motivation and practical advice for you as you work toward greater health.

TABLE OF CONTENT

TABLE OF CONTENT

TABLE OF CONTENT

Turmeric Latte
Pineapple Ginger Juice
Cucumber Mint Cooler
Green Tea with Turmeric and Ginger
Blueberry Kombucha
Mango Turmeric Smoothie
Tart Cherry Juice
Aloe Vera Juice
Pomegranate Juice with Ginger
Green Juice with Wheatgrass and Spinach
Apple Cider Vinegar and Honey Drink
Golden Milk with Cinnamon and Cardamom
Carrot and Ginger Juice
Hibiscus and Orange Iced Tea
Cucumber and Lime Infused Water
Cranberry and Orange Juice
Watermelon and Mint Smoothie
Ginger and Lemon Tea with Honey
Sweet Potato and Carrot Juice with Ginger
Pineapple and Ginger Juice
Mango and Ginger Iced Tea
Lemon and Ginger Turmeric Tonic
Cinnamon and Honey Hot Cocoa

TABLE OF CONTENT

Why You Need a Stomach Ulcer Diet Cookbook

If you or someone you know has been diagnosed with a stomach ulcer, and you're probably asking, "Why do I need a stomach ulcer diet cookbook?" Let me tell you, having a stomach ulcer may be a real pain in the gut.

A stomach ulcer is a sore that develops in the lining of your stomach or small intestine and may cause severe pain, bloating, nausea, and vomiting. Following a stomach ulcer diet is one method to control your symptoms and accelerate recovery.

A stomach ulcer diet consists of eating meals that may help calm and mend your stomach lining while avoiding foods that might worsen your ulcer. A stomach ulcer diet cookbook might be useful in this situation.

You may find a broad variety of meals in a cookbook that is specifically designed for someone on a stomach ulcer diet. These dishes are created to be simple to digest while yet giving your body the nutrition it needs to repair and recover.

These are some of the reasons why you should purchase a stomach ulcer diet cookbook:

Variety: You may pick from a wide selection of dishes in a stomach ulcer diet cookbook. This keeps you from becoming bored and makes it simpler for you to follow your diet.

Why You Need a Stomach Ulcer Diet Cookbook

Convenience: Finding meals that are safe to consume might be challenging if you have a stomach ulcer. You won't need to spend hours looking through menus to locate meals that are suitable for your requirements if you have a stomach ulcer diet cookbook.

Has all the key vitamins and minerals your body needs to heal and recover. Nutrient-dense: Recipes in a stomach ulcer diet cookbook are created to be nutrient-dense.

Healing characteristics: Some of the foods in a diet for stomach ulcers, such honey, garlic, and ginger, have been demonstrated to have healing effects. You may use recipes from a cookbook on the stomach ulcer diet to help you boost healing and lower inflammation.

Advice from experts: Numerous cookbooks on the stomach ulcer diet are produced by professionals in the fields of nutrition and digestive health. These professionals provide you insightful guidance on how to control your symptoms and encourage recovery.

Introduction

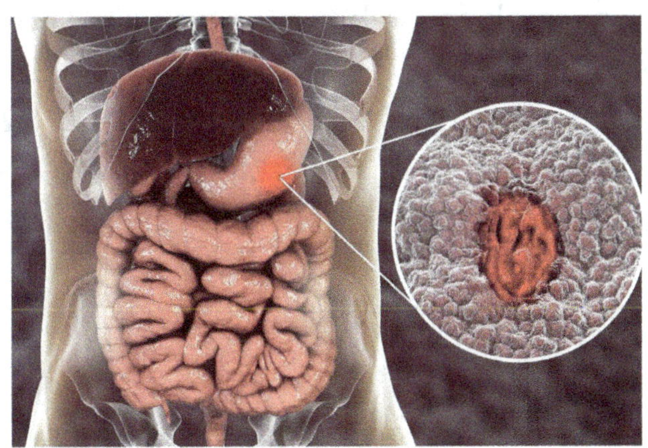

Do you struggle to eat your favorite meals without thinking about the agony and anguish you could experience due to stomach ulcers? Worry no more! In addition to soothing your stomach, our new cookbook will help you enjoy scrumptious smoothies and beverages that will also provide the nutrients you need to stay healthy and satisfied.

We have a collection of drinks in our cookbook that are

targeted towards stomach ulcers and recovery. Every recipe, from fruity smoothies to hot ginger beverages, is painstakingly created with the ideal combination of ingredients to help you manage your symptoms and enhance your general health. While having stomach ulcers might be very difficult, we think that eating should never be a burden.

We've prepared this cookbook to help you enjoy your favorite tastes while still looking after your stomach. Our cookbook thus contains everything you need, whether you're searching for a quick and simple morning smoothie or a cool drink to enjoy on a hot summer day. Wave goodbye to boring, bland meals and welcome to a new world of enticing, therapeutic smoothies and beverages!

Be ready to go on a journey to a healthy and happy life as you discover a whole new world of delights. Drink to good health with me!

Chapter 1

SMOOTHIES FOR STOMACH ULCERS

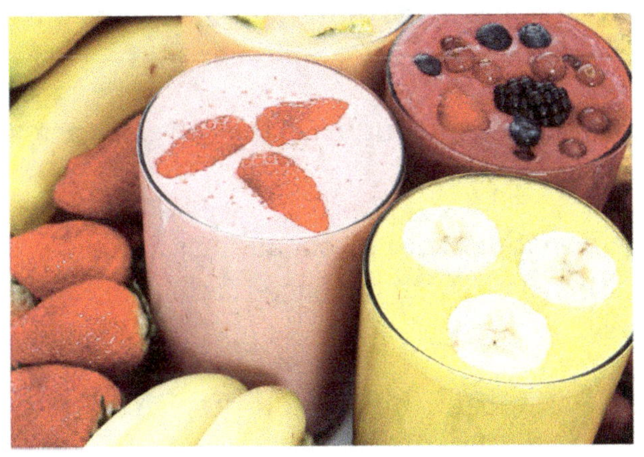

BANANA OAT SMOOTHIE

Ingredients:

- 1 ripe banana, peeled and sliced
- 1/2 cup old-fashioned rolled oats
- 1 cup unsweetened almond milk
- 1/4 cup plain Greek yogurt
- 1 tablespoon honey
- 1/4 teaspoon ground cinnamon
- 4-5 ice cubes

1) In a blender, combine the banana, rolled oats, almond milk, Greek yogurt, honey, and ground cinnamon.
2) Add the ice cubes and blend until smooth.
3) Pour into a glass and enjoy immediately.

Notes:

•You can use any type of milk you prefer, but almond milk is a good option for people with stomach ulcers as it is lower in fat and lactose compared to cow's milk.

•Greek yogurt is also a good option as it is lower in lactose compared to regular yogurt.

•Honey can help soothe a sore throat and has antibacterial properties that may help fight the bacteria that can cause stomach ulcers.

•Cinnamon is a natural anti-inflammatory spice that can help soothe stomach inflammation.

•If you find that the smoothie is too thick, you can add more almond milk or water to thin it out.

BLUEBERRY ALMOND SMOOTHIE

Ingredients:

- 1 cup frozen blueberries
- 1/2 cup unsweetened almond milk
- 1/4 cup plain Greek yogurt
- 1/4 cup sliced almonds
- 1 tablespoon honey

- 4-5 ice cubes

Mixing Guidelines:

1) In a blender, combine the frozen blueberries, almond milk, Greek yogurt, sliced almonds, and honey.
2) Add the ice cubes and blend until smooth.
3) Pour into a glass.

PAPAYA GINGER SMOOTHIE

Ingredients:

- 1 ripe papaya, peeled and chopped
- 1 banana, peeled and sliced
- 1 cup plain Greek yogurt
- 1/2 cup unsweetened almond milk
- 1 tbsp freshly grated ginger
- 1 tbsp honey
- 1/2 cup ice

Mixing Guidelines:

1) Add the chopped papaya, sliced banana, Greek yogurt, unsweetened almond milk, freshly grated ginger, and honey to a blender.
2) Blend the ingredients until smooth.
3) Add ice and blend again until the mixture is thick and creamy.
4) Taste the smoothie and adjust the sweetness by adding more honey if desired.
5) Pour the smoothie into a glass.

PINEAPPLE BANANA SMOOTHIE

Ingredients:

- 1 cup frozen pineapple chunks
- 1 ripe banana, peeled and sliced
- 1 cup unsweetened coconut milk
- 1/2 cup plain Greek yogurt
- 1 tbsp honey
- 1/2 tsp vanilla extract
- 1/2 cup ice

Mixing Guidelines:

1) Add the frozen pineapple chunks, sliced banana, unsweetened coconut milk, plain Greek yogurt, honey, and vanilla extract to a blender.
2) Blend the ingredients until smooth.
3) Add ice and blend again until the mixture is thick and creamy.
4) Taste the smoothie and adjust the sweetness by adding more honey if desired.
5) Pour the smoothie into a glass

MANGO YOGURT SMOOTHIE

Ingredients:

- 1 ripe mango, peeled and chopped
- 1 cup plain Greek yogurt
- 1/2 cup unsweetened almond milk
- 1 tbsp. honey

- 1/2 tsp vanilla extract
- 1/2 cup ice

Mixing Guidelines:

1) Add the chopped mango, plain Greek yogurt, unsweetened almond milk, honey, and vanilla extract to a blender.
2) Blend the ingredients until smooth.
3) Add ice and blend again until the mixture is thick and creamy.
4) Taste the smoothie and adjust the sweetness by adding more honey if desired.
5) Pour the smoothie into a glass

SPINACH BERRY SMOOTHIE

Ingredients:

- 1 cup fresh spinach leaves
- 1/2 cup frozen mixed berries
- 1/2 banana, sliced
- 1/2 cup plain Greek yogurt
- 1/2 cup unsweetened almond milk
- 1 tsp honey (optional)
- 1/2 cup ice cubes

Mixing Guidelines:

1) Add the fresh spinach leaves, frozen mixed berries, sliced banana, plain Greek yogurt, unsweetened almond milk, and honey (optional) to a blender.
2) Blend the ingredients until smooth.

3) Add ice cubes and blend again until the mixture is thick and creamy.
4) Taste the smoothie and adjust the sweetness by adding more honey if desired.
5) Pour the smoothie into a glass

PEACH ALMOND SMOOTHIE

Ingredients:

- 1 ripe peach, pitted and sliced
- 1/4 cup raw almonds
- 1/2 cup plain Greek yogurt
- 1/2 cup unsweetened almond milk
- 1 tsp honey (optional)
- 1/2 tsp vanilla extract
- 1/2 cup ice cubes

Mixing Guidelines:

1) Add the sliced peach, raw almonds, plain Greek yogurt, unsweetened almond milk, honey (optional), and vanilla extract to a blender.
2) Blend the ingredients until smooth.
3) Add ice cubes and blend again until the mixture is thick and creamy.
4) Taste the smoothie and adjust the sweetness by adding more honey if desired.
5) Pour the smoothie into a glass

CARROT ORANGE SMOOTHIE

- 2 medium-sized carrots, peeled and chopped
- 1 large orange, peeled and seeded
- 1/2 banana, sliced
- 1/2 cup plain Greek yogurt
- 1/2 cup unsweetened almond milk
- 1 tsp honey (optional)
- 1/2 tsp grated ginger (optional)
- 1/2 cup ice cubes

Mixing Guidelines:

1) Add the chopped carrots, orange segments, sliced banana, plain Greek yogurt, unsweetened almond milk, honey (optional), and grated ginger (optional) to a blender.
2) Blend the ingredients until smooth.
3) Add ice cubes and blend again until the mixture is thick and creamy
4) Taste the smoothie and adjust the sweetness by adding more honey if desired.
5) Pour the smoothie into a glass

COCONUT MANGO SMOOTHIE

Ingredients:

- 1 ripe mango, peeled and chopped
- 1/2 cup coconut milk
- 1/2 cup plain Greek yogurt
- 1/2 cup unsweetened almond milk
- 1 tsp honey (optional)

- 1/2 tsp vanilla extract
- 1/2 cup ice cubes

Mixing Guidelines:

1) Add the chopped mango, coconut milk, plain Greek yogurt, unsweetened almond milk, honey (optional), and vanilla extract to a blender.
2) Blend the ingredients until smooth.
3) Add ice cubes and blend again until the mixture is thick and creamy.
4) Taste the smoothie and adjust the sweetness by adding more honey if desired.
5) Pour the smoothie into a glass

BLUEBERRY BANANA SMOOTHIE WITH FLAXSEED

Ingredients:

- 1 ripe banana, sliced
- 1/2 cup frozen blueberries
- 1/2 cup plain Greek yogurt
- 1/2 cup unsweetened almond milk
- 1 tbsp ground flaxseed
- 1 tsp honey (optional)
- 1/2 cup ice cubes

Mixing Guidelines:

1) Add the sliced banana, frozen blueberries, plain Greek yogurt, unsweetened almond milk, ground flaxseed, and honey (optional) to a blender.

2) Blend the ingredients until smooth.

3) Add ice cubes and blend again until the mixture is thick and creamy.

4) Taste the smoothie and adjust the sweetness by adding more honey if desired.

5) Pour the smoothie into a glass

GREEN APPLE SMOOTHIE WITH CINNAMON

Ingredients:

- 1 green apple, cored and chopped
- 1/2 banana, sliced
- 1/2 cup plain Greek yogurt
- 1/2 cup unsweetened almond milk
- 1 tsp honey (optional)
- 1/2 tsp ground cinnamon
- 1/2 cup ice cubes

Mixing Guidelines:

1) Add the chopped green apple, sliced banana, plain Greek yogurt, unsweetened almond milk, honey (optional), and ground cinnamon to a blender.

2) Blend the ingredients until smooth.

3) Add ice cubes and blend again until the mixture is thick and creamy.

4) Taste the smoothie and adjust the sweetness by adding more honey if desired.

5) Pour the smoothie into a glass

BLACKBERRY GINGER SMOOTHIE

Ingredients:

- 1 cup fresh blackberries
- 1 inch piece of fresh ginger, peeled and chopped
- 1/2 cup plain Greek yogurt
- 1/2 cup unsweetened almond milk
- 1 tsp honey (optional)
- 1/2 tsp vanilla extract
- 1/2 cup ice cubes

Mixing Guidelines:

1) Add the fresh blackberries, chopped ginger, plain Greek yogurt, unsweetened almond milk, honey (optional), and vanilla extract to a blender.
2) Blend the ingredients until smooth.
3) Add ice cubes and blend again until the mixture is thick and creamy.
4) Taste the smoothie and adjust the sweetness by adding more honey if desired.
5) Pour the smoothie into a glass

HONEYDEW MELON SMOOTHIE WITH MINT

Ingredients:

- 2 cups chopped honeydew melon
- 1/2 cup plain Greek yogurt
- 1/2 cup unsweetened coconut milk
- 1 tsp honey (optional)

- 1/4 cup fresh mint leaves
- 1/2 cup ice cubes

Mixing Guidelines:

1) Add the chopped honeydew melon, plain Greek yogurt, unsweetened coconut milk, honey (optional), and fresh mint leaves to a blender.
2) Blend the ingredients until smooth.
3) Add ice cubes and blend again until the mixture is thick and creamy.
4) Taste the smoothie and adjust the sweetness by adding more honey if desired
5) Pour the smoothie into a glass

KIWI PINEAPPLE SMOOTHIE

Ingredients:

- 2 kiwis, peeled and chopped
- 1 cup chopped fresh pineapple
- 1/2 banana, sliced
- 1/2 cup unsweetened almond milk
- 1/2 cup plain Greek yogurt
- 1 tsp honey (optional)
- 1/2 cup ice cubes

Mixing Guidelines:

1) Add the chopped kiwis, chopped pineapple, sliced banana, unsweetened almond milk, plain Greek yogurt, and honey (optional) to a blender.
2) Blend the ingredients until smooth.

3) Add ice cubes and blend again until the mixture is thick and creamy.
4) Taste the smoothie and adjust the sweetness by adding more honey if desired.
5) Pour the smoothie into a glass

SWEET POTATO SMOOTHIE WITH CINNAMON

Ingredients:

- 1 small sweet potato, cooked and peeled
- 1/2 banana, sliced
- 1/2 cup unsweetened almond milk
- 1/2 cup plain Greek yogurt
- 1 tsp honey (optional)
- 1/2 tsp ground cinnamon
- 1/2 tsp vanilla extract
- 1/2 cup ice cubes

Mixing Guidelines:

1) Add the cooked and peeled sweet potato, sliced banana, unsweetened almond milk, plain Greek yogurt, honey (optional), ground cinnamon, and vanilla extract to a blender.
2) Blend the ingredients until smooth.
3) Add ice cubes and blend again until the mixture is thick and creamy.
4) Taste the smoothie and adjust the sweetness by adding more honey if desired.
5) Pour the smoothie into a glass

CHERRY VANILLA SMOOTHIE

Ingredients:

- 1 cup frozen cherries
- 1/2 banana, sliced
- 1/2 cup unsweetened almond milk
- 1/2 cup plain Greek yogurt
- 1 tsp honey (optional)
- 1/2 tsp vanilla extract
- 1/2 cup ice cubes

Mixing Guidelines:

1) Add the frozen cherries, sliced banana, unsweetened almond milk, plain Greek yogurt, honey (optional), and vanilla extract to a blender.
2) Blend the ingredients until smooth.
3) Add ice cubes and blend again until the mixture is thick and creamy.
4) Taste the smoothie and adjust the sweetness by adding more honey if desired.
5) Pour the smoothie into a glass

PEAR GINGER SMOOTHIE

Ingredients:

- 1 ripe pear, peeled and chopped
- 1/2 banana, sliced
- 1/2 cup unsweetened almond milk
- 1/2 cup plain Greek yogurt

- 1 tsp honey (optional)
- 1 tsp grated ginger
- 1/2 tsp vanilla extract
- 1/2 cup ice cubes

Mixing Guidelines:

1) Add the chopped pear, sliced banana, unsweetened almond milk, plain Greek yogurt, honey (optional), grated ginger, and vanilla extract to a blender.
2) Blend the ingredients until smooth.
3) Add ice cubes and blend again until the mixture is thick and creamy.
4) Taste the smoothie and adjust the sweetness by adding more honey if desired.
5) Pour the smoothie into a glass

PUMPKIN SMOOTHIE WITH NUTMEG

Ingredients:

- 1/2 cup pumpkin puree
- 1/2 banana, sliced
- 1/2 cup unsweetened almond milk
- 1/2 cup plain Greek yogurt
- 1 tsp honey (optional)
- 1/2 tsp ground nutmeg
- 1/2 tsp cinnamon
- 1/2 tsp vanilla extract
- 1/2 cup ice cubes

1) Add the pumpkin puree, sliced banana, unsweetened almond milk, plain Greek yogurt, honey (optional), ground nutmeg, cinnamon, and vanilla extract to a blender.
2) Blend the ingredients until smooth.
3) Add ice cubes and blend again until the mixture is thick and creamy.
4) Taste the smoothie and adjust the sweetness by adding more honey if desired.
5) Pour the smoothie into a glass and sprinkle with additional cinnamon.

BEETROOT AND CARROT SMOOTHIE

Ingredients:

- 1 small beetroot, peeled and chopped
- 1 large carrot, peeled and chopped
- 1/2 cup unsweetened almond milk
- 1/2 cup plain Greek yogurt
- 1 tsp honey (optional)
- 1/2 tsp ginger powder
- 1/2 tsp cinnamon
- 1/2 tsp vanilla extract
- 1/2 cup ice cubes

Mixing Guidelines:

1) Add the chopped beetroot, chopped carrot, unsweetened almond milk, plain Greek yogurt, honey (optional), ginger powder, cinnamon, and vanilla

extract to a blender.

2) Blend the ingredients until smooth.

3) Add ice cubes and blend again until the mixture is thick and creamy.

4) Taste the smoothie and adjust the sweetness by adding more honey if desired.

5) Pour the smoothie into a glass

WATERMELON MINT SMOOTHIE

Ingredients:

- 2 cups chopped watermelon, seeds removed
- 1/2 cup unsweetened coconut milk
- 1/2 cup plain Greek yogurt
- 1 tsp honey (optional)
- 1/4 cup fresh mint leaves
- 1/2 cup ice cubes

Mixing Guidelines:

1) Add the chopped watermelon, unsweetened coconut milk, plain Greek yogurt, honey (optional), and fresh mint leaves to a blender.

2) Blend the ingredients until smooth.

3) Add ice cubes and blend again until the mixture is thick and creamy.

4) Taste the smoothie and adjust the sweetness by adding more honey if desired.

5) Pour the smoothie into a glass and garnish with additional fresh mint leaves.

CHOCOLATE PEANUT BUTTER SMOOTHIE

Ingredients:

- 1 banana, peeled and frozen
- 1 cup unsweetened almond milk
- 1/4 cup creamy peanut butter
- 2 tbsp unsweetened cocoa powder
- 1 tbsp honey (optional)
- 1/2 tsp vanilla extract
- 1/2 cup ice cubes

Mixing Guidelines:

1) Add the frozen banana, unsweetened almond milk, creamy peanut butter, unsweetened cocoa powder, honey (optional), and vanilla extract to a blender.
2) Blend the ingredients until smooth.
3) Add ice cubes and blend again until the mixture is thick and creamy.
4) Taste the smoothie and adjust the sweetness by adding more honey if desired.
5) Pour the smoothie into a glass

STRAWBERRY COCONUT MILK SMOOTHIE

Ingredients:

- 1 cup frozen strawberries
- 1 cup unsweetened coconut milk
- 1/2 banana
- 1/2 tsp vanilla extract

- 1 tsp honey (optional)
- 1/2 cup ice cubes

Mixing Guidelines:

1) Add the frozen strawberries, unsweetened coconut milk, banana, vanilla extract, and honey (optional) to a blender.
2) Blend the ingredients until smooth.
3) Add ice cubes and blend again until the mixture is thick and creamy.
4) Taste the smoothie and adjust the sweetness by adding more honey if desired.
5) Pour the smoothie into a glass

RASPBERRY PEACH SMOOTHIE

Ingredients:

- 1 cup frozen raspberries
- 1 ripe peach, pitted and chopped
- 1/2 cup unsweetened almond milk
- 1/2 cup plain Greek yogurt
- 1 tsp honey (optional)
- 1/2 cup ice cubes

Mixing Guidelines:

1) Add the frozen raspberries, chopped peach, unsweetened almond milk, plain Greek yogurt, and honey (optional) to a blender.
2) Blend the ingredients until smooth.
3) Add ice cubes and blend again until the mixture is

thick and creamy.
4) Taste the smoothie and adjust the sweetness by adding more honey if desired.
5) Pour the smoothie into a glass

TEA FOR STOMACH ULCERS

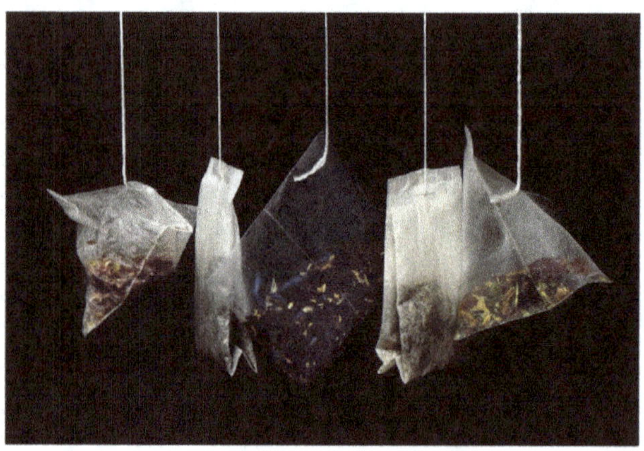

CHAMOMILE TEA

Ingredients:

- 1 chamomile tea bag or 1 tablespoon dried chamomile flowers
- 8 ounces of water
- Honey or lemon, to taste (optional)

Mixing Guidelines:

1) Boil 8 ounces of water in a tea kettle or on the stove.
2) Place a chamomile tea bag or 1 tablespoon of dried chamomile flowers into a tea infuser or a tea strainer.
3) Place the tea infuser or tea strainer into a cup or mug.
4) Pour the hot water over the chamomile tea bag or flowers.
5) Let the tea steep for 5-10 minutes.
6) Remove the tea bag or strainer and discard.
7) If desired, add honey or lemon to taste.

LICORICE ROOT TEA

Ingredients:

- 1 licorice root tea bag or 1 tablespoon of dried licorice root
- 8 ounces of water
- Honey, to taste (optional)

Mixing Guidelines:

1) Boil 8 ounces of water in a tea kettle or on the stove.
2) Place a licorice root tea bag or 1 tablespoon of dried licorice root into a tea infuser or a tea strainer.
3) Place the tea infuser or tea strainer into a cup or mug.
4) Pour the hot water over the licorice root tea bag or root.
5) Let the tea steep for 5-10 minutes
6) Remove the tea bag or strainer and discard.
7) If desired, add honey to taste.

GINGER TEA

Ingredients:

- 1 inch fresh ginger root, peeled and sliced
- 8-10 ounces of water
- Honey or lemon, to taste (optional)

Mixing Guidelines:

1) Bring 8-10 ounces of water to a boil in a tea kettle or on the stove.
2) Peel and slice 1 inch of fresh ginger root
3) Place the sliced ginger into a tea infuser or a tea strainer.
4) Place the tea infuser or tea strainer into a cup or mug.
5) Pour the hot water over the sliced ginger.
6) Let the tea steep for 5-10 minutes.
7) Remove the tea infuser or strainer and discard the ginger.
8) If desired, add honey or lemon to taste.

FENNEL TEA

Ingredients:

- 1 tablespoon of fennel seeds
- 8-10 ounces of water
- Honey or lemon, to taste (optional)

Mixing Guidelines:

1) Bring 8-10 ounces of water to a boil in a tea kettle or on the stove.
2) Add 1 tablespoon of fennel seeds to the hot water.
3) Reduce the heat to low and let the tea simmer for 5-10 minutes
4) Remove the pot from the heat and let the tea steep for an additional 5-10 minutes.
5) Strain the tea using a fine-mesh strainer.
6) If desired, add honey or lemon to taste.

MARSHMALLOW ROOT TEA

Ingredients:

- 1 tablespoon of dried marshmallow root
- 8-10 ounces of water
- Honey or lemon, to taste (optional)

Mixing Guidelines:

1) Bring 8-10 ounces of water to a boil in a tea kettle or on the stove.
2) Add 1 tablespoon of dried marshmallow root to the hot water.
3) Reduce the heat to low and let the tea simmer for 5-10 minutes.
4) Remove the pot from the heat and let the tea steep for an additional 5-10 minutes.
5) Strain the tea using a fine-mesh strainer.
6) If desired, add honey or lemon to taste.

PEPPERMINT TEA

Ingredients:

- 1-2 peppermint tea bags OR 1-2 tablespoons of dried peppermint leaves
- 8-10 ounces of water
- Honey or lemon, to taste (optional)

Mixing Guidelines:

1) Bring 8-10 ounces of water to a boil in a tea kettle or on the stove.
2) Place 1-2 peppermint tea bags OR 1-2 tablespoons of dried peppermint leaves in a mug.
3) Pour the hot water over the tea bags or leaves.
4) Let the tea steep for 3-5 minutes.
5) Remove the tea bags or strain the tea using a fine-mesh strainer if using loose leaves.
6) If desired, add honey or lemon to taste.

LEMON BALM TEA

Ingredients:

- 1-2 lemon balm tea bags OR 1-2 tablespoons of dried lemon balm leaves
- 8-10 ounces of water
- Honey or lemon, to taste (optional)

Mixing Guidelines:

1) Bring 8-10 ounces of water to a boil in a tea kettle or on the stove.
2) Place 1-2 lemon balm tea bags OR 1-2 tablespoons of dried lemon balm leaves in a mug.
3) Pour the hot water over the tea bags or leaves.
4) Let the tea steep for 5-10 minutes.
5) Remove the tea bags or strain the tea using a fine-mesh strainer if using loose leaves.
6) If desired, add honey or lemon to taste.

SLIPPERY ELM TEA

Ingredients:

- 1-2 tablespoons of slippery elm bark powder
- 8-10 ounces of water
- Honey or lemon, to taste (optional)

Mixing Guidelines:

1) Bring 8-10 ounces of water to a boil in a tea kettle or on the stove.
2) Place 1-2 tablespoons of slippery elm bark powder in a mug.
3) Pour the hot water over the slippery elm bark powder.
4) Whisk the mixture vigorously with a fork or small whisk until the slippery elm powder is fully dissolved.
5) Let the tea steep for 3-5 minutes.
6) If desired, add honey or lemon to taste.

RASPBERRY LEAF TEA

- 1-2 teaspoons of dried raspberry leaves (or a handful of fresh leaves)
- 2 cups of water
- Honey or stevia (optional)

Mixing Guidelines:

1) Boil the water in a pot on the stove.
2) Once the water has reached boiling point, remove it from the heat and add the raspberry leaves.
3) Allow the leaves to steep in the water for about 10-15 minutes.
4) Strain the tea into a cup or teapot.
5) Add honey or stevia to taste, if desired.

ECHINACEA TEA

Ingredients:

- 1-2 teaspoons of dried Echinacea leaves or flowers
- 2 cups of water
- Honey or stevia (optional)

Mixing Guidelines:

1) Boil the water in a pot on the stove.
2) Once the water has reached boiling point, remove it from the heat and add the Echinacea leaves or flowers.

3) Allow the Echinacea to steep in the water for about 10-15 minutes.
4) Strain the tea into a cup or teapot.
5) Add honey or stevia to taste, if desired.

CALENDULA TEA

Ingredients:

- 1-2 teaspoons of dried Calendula flowers
- 2 cups of water
- Honey or stevia (optional)

Mixing Guidelines:

1) Boil the water in a pot on the stove.
2) Once the water has reached boiling point, remove it from the heat and add the Calendula flowers.
3) Allow the Calendula to steep in the water for about 10-15 minutes.
4) Strain the tea into a cup or teapot.
5) Add honey or stevia to taste, if desired.

LAVENDER TEA

Ingredients:

- 1-2 teaspoons of dried lavender buds
- 2 cups of water
- Honey or stevia (optional)

Mixing Guidelines:

1) Boil the water in a pot on the stove.
2) Once the water has reached boiling point, remove it from the heat and add the lavender buds.
3) Allow the lavender to steep in the water for about 5-7 minutes.
4) Strain the tea into a cup or teapot
5) Add honey or stevia to taste, if desired.

SAGE TEA

Ingredients:

- 1-2 teaspoons of dried sage leaves
- 2 cups of water
- Honey or stevia (optional)

Mixing Guidelines:

1) Boil the water in a pot on the stove.
2) Once the water has reached boiling point, remove it from the heat and add the sage leaves.
3) Allow the sage to steep in the water for about 10-15 minutes.
4) Strain the tea into a cup or teapot.
5) Add honey or stevia to taste, if desired.

DANDELION ROOT TEA

Ingredients:

- 1-2 teaspoons of dried dandelion root
- 2 cups of water
  Honey or stevia (optional)

Mixing Guidelines:

1) Boil the water in a pot on the stove.
2) Once the water has reached boiling point, remove it from the heat and add the dandelion root
3) Allow the dandelion root to steep in the water for about 10-15 minutes.
4) Strain the tea into a cup or teapot.
5) Add honey or stevia to taste, if desired.

NETTLE TEA

Ingredients:

- 1-2 teaspoons of dried nettle leaves
- 2 cups of water
- Honey or stevia (optional)

Mixing Guidelines:

1) Boil the water in a pot on the stove.
2) Once the water has reached boiling point, remove it from the heat and add the nettle leaves.
3) Allow the nettle leaves to steep in the water for about 5-7 minutcs.
4) Strain the tea into a cup or teapot.
5) Add honey or stevia to taste, if desired.

HIBISCUS TEA

Ingredients:

- 1-2 teaspoons of dried hibiscus flowers
- 2 cups of water
- Honey or stevia (optional)

Mixing Guidelines:

1) Boil the water in a pot on the stove.
2) Once the water has reached boiling point, remove it from the heat and add the hibiscus flowers.
3) Allow the hibiscus flowers to steep in the water for about 5-7 minutes.
4) Strain the tea into a cup or teapot.
5) Add honey or stevia to taste, if desired.

LEMON VERBENA TEA

Ingredients:

- 1-2 teaspoons of dried lemon verbena leaves
- 2 cups of water
- Honey or stevia (optional)

Mixing Guidelines:

1) Boil the water in a pot on the stove.
2) Once the water has reached boiling point, remove it from the heat and add the lemon verbena leaves.
3) Allow the lemon verbena leaves to steep in the water for about 5-7 minutes.

4) Strain the tea into a cup or teapot.
5) Add honey or stevia to taste, if desired.

ROSE HIP TEA

Ingredients:

- 1-2 teaspoons of dried rose hips
- 2 cups of water
- Honey or stevia (optional)

Mixing Guidelines:

1) Boil the water in a pot on the stove.
2) Once the water has reached boiling point, remove it from the heat and add the dried rose hips.
3) Allow the rose hips to steep in the water for about 5-7 minutes.
4) Strain the tea into a cup or teapot.
5) Add honey or stevia to taste, if desired.

ASTRAGALUS TEA

Ingredients:

- 1-2 teaspoons of dried astragalus root
- 2 cups of water
- Honey or stevia (optional)

Mixing Guidelines:

1) Rinse the dried astragalus root in cold water to

remove any dirt or impurities.

2) Add the astragalus root to a pot with 2 cups of water.
3) Bring the water to a boil, then reduce the heat and let the tea simmer for 15-20 minutes.
4) Remove the pot from the heat and let the tea steep for an additional 5-10 minutes.
5) Strain the tea into a cup or teapot
6) Add honey or stevia to taste, if desired.

CATNIP TEA

Ingredients:

- 1-2 teaspoons of dried catnip leaves and flowers
- 2 cups of water
- Honey or stevia (optional)

Mixing Guidelines:

1) Boil the water in a pot on the stove.
2) Once the water has reached boiling point, remove it from the heat and add the dried catnip leaves and flowers.
3) Allow the catnip to steep in the water for about 5-7 minutes.
4) Strain the tea into a cup or teapot.
5) Add honey or stevia to taste, if desired.

PASSIONFLOWER TEA

Ingredients:

- 1-2 teaspoons of dried passionflower leaves, flowers, and stems
- 2 cups of water
- Honey or stevia (optional)

Mixing Guidelines:

1) Boil the water in a pot on the stove.
2) Once the water has reached boiling point, remove it from the heat and add the dried passionflower leaves, flowers, and stems.
3) Allow the passionflower to steep in the water for about 5-7 minutes.
4) Strain the tea into a cup or teapot
5) Add honey or stevia to taste, if desired.

CHAMOMILE AND LAVENDER TEA

Ingredients:

- 1-2 teaspoons of dried chamomile flowers
- 1-2 teaspoons of dried lavender buds
- 2 cups of water
- Honey or stevia (optional)

Mixing Guidelines:

1) Boil the water in a pot on the stove.
2) Once the water has reached boiling point, remove it from the heat and add the dried chamomile flowers and lavender buds.
3) Allow the herbs to steep in the water for about 5-7 minutes.

4) Strain the tea into a cup or teapot.
5) Add honey or stevia to taste, if desired.

LEMONGRASS AND GINGER TEA

Ingredients:

- 1-2 stalks of dried lemongrass (or 1-2 teaspoons of dried lemongrass)
- 1-2 inches of fresh ginger root, peeled and sliced
- 2 cups of water
- Honey or stevia (optional)

Mixing Guidelines:

1) Boil the water in a pot on the stove.
2) Once the water has reached boiling point, remove it from the heat and add the dried lemongrass and fresh ginger slices.
3) Allow the herbs to steep in the water for about 5-7 minutes.
4) Strain the tea into a cup or teapot.
5) Add honey or stevia to taste, if desired.

Chapter 3

ANTI-INFLAMMATORY FOR STOMACH ULCERS

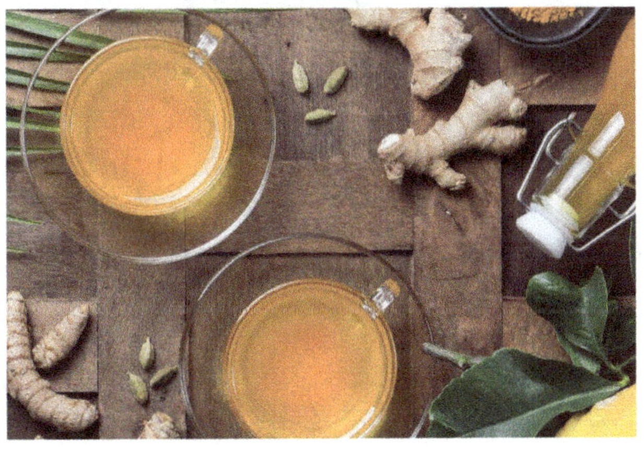

TURMERIC LATTE

Ingredients:

- 1 cup of unsweetened almond milk (or any milk of

your choice)

- 1 teaspoon of ground turmeric
- 1/2 teaspoon of ground cinnamon
- 1/4 teaspoon of ground ginger
- 1/4 teaspoon of ground cardamom
- 1-2 teaspoons of honey or maple syrup (optional)

Mixing Guidelines:

1) In a small pot, heat the almond milk over medium heat until it starts to steam.
2) Add the ground turmeric, cinnamon, ginger, and cardamom to the pot, and whisk to combine.
3) Continue to heat the mixture for 2-3 minutes, whisking occasionally, until the spices are fragrant and the mixture is heated through.
4) Remove the pot from the heat and pour the latte into a mug.
5) Add honey or maple syrup to taste, if desired.

PINEAPPLE GINGER JUICE

Ingredients:

- 1/2 a pineapple, peeled and chopped
- 1-2 inches of fresh ginger root, peeled and sliced
- 1 cup of water
- Honey or stevia (optional)

Mixing Guidelines:

1) Add the chopped pineapple and sliced ginger to a blender.

2) Add 1 cup of water to the blender, and blend until the mixture is smooth.
3) Strain the mixture through a fine-mesh strainer or cheesecloth to remove any pulp.
4) Pour the juice into a glass.
5) Add honey or stevia to taste, if desired.

CUCUMBER MINT COOLER

Ingredients:

- 1 large cucumber, peeled and chopped
- 1/4 cup of fresh mint leaves
- 1 cup of water
- Juice of 1/2 a lemon
- Honey or stevia (optional)
- Ice cubes

Mixing Guidelines:

1) Add the chopped cucumber and mint leaves to a blender.
2) Add 1 cup of water to the blender, and blend until the mixture is smooth.
3) Strain the mixture through a fine-mesh strainer or cheesecloth to remove any pulp.
4) Add the lemon juice to the strained mixture and stir.
5) Pour the mixture into a glass filled with ice cubes.
6) Add honey or stevia to taste, if desired.

GREEN TEA WITH TURMERIC AND GINGER

- 1 green tea bag
- 1/2 teaspoon ground turmeric
- 1/2 teaspoon ground ginger
- 2 cups of water
- Honey or stevia (optional)

Mixing Guidelines:

1) Add 2 cups of water to a small pot and bring it to a boil.
2) Reduce the heat to low, and add the green tea bag, ground turmeric, and ground ginger to the pot.
3) Let the mixture simmer for 2-3 minutes.
4) Remove the pot from the heat and let the mixture steep for another 2-3 minutes.
5) Remove the tea bag from the pot, and pour the tea into a mug.
6) Add honey or stevia to taste, if desired.

BLUEBERRY KOMBUCHA

Ingredients:

- 1 cup of fresh or frozen blueberries
- 1/2 cup of white sugar
- 4 black tea bags
- 1 scoby (symbiotic culture of bacteria and yeast)
- 1 cup of kombucha from a previous batch
- 3 quarts of filtered water

* Glass jars with lids

Mixing Guidelines:

1) Bring 3 quarts of filtered water to a boil in a large pot.
2) Add 4 black tea bags to the pot and let it steep for 5-10 minutes.
3) Remove the tea bags from the pot and stir in 1/2 cup of white sugar until it dissolves.
4) Let the tea mixture cool to room temperature.
5) Add the cooled tea mixture to a glass jar and add 1 cup of kombucha from a previous batch.
6) Place a scoby on top of the liquid, and cover the jar with a lid or a breathable cloth.
7) Store the jar in a warm, dark place for 7-10 days, until the kombucha has fermented to your desired taste.
8) Once the kombucha has fermented, remove the scoby and 1 cup of the kombucha for a future batch.
9) Add 1 cup of fresh or frozen blueberries to the jar and let it sit for an additional 1-2 days to infuse the blueberry flavor into the kombucha.
10) Once the blueberry flavor has infused, strain the kombucha into glass jars, and store them in the fridge until ready to serve.

MANGO TURMERIC SMOOTHIE

Ingredients:

* 1 cup frozen mango chunks
* 1 small banana
* 1 tsp ground turmeric
* 1 tsp grated fresh ginger

- 1/2 cup unsweetened almond milk
- 1/2 cup plain Greek yogurt
- 1 tsp honey (optional)

Mixing Guidelines:

1) Add the frozen mango chunks, banana, turmeric, ginger, almond milk, Greek yogurt, and honey (if using) to a blender.
2) Blend the ingredients until smooth and creamy.
3) Pour the smoothie into a glass.

TART CHERRY JUICE

Ingredients:

- 2 cups of fresh or frozen tart cherries
- 2 cups of water
- Honey or other natural sweeteners (optional)

Mixing Guidelines:

1) Rinse the tart cherries and remove the stems and pits.
2) Add the cherries and water to a blender and blend until smooth.
3) Pour the mixture through a strainer or cheesecloth to remove any pulp or solids.
4) Taste the juice and add honey or other natural sweeteners if desired.
5) Chill the juice in the fridge for at least 30 minutes before serving.

ALOE VERA JUICE

Ingredients:

- 1 large aloe vera leaf
- 2 cups of water
- Honey or other natural sweeteners (optional)
- Lemon juice (optional)

Mixing Guidelines:

1) Rinse the aloe vera leaf and cut off the spiky edges.
2) Slice the leaf open lengthwise and scoop out the clear gel inside using a spoon.
3) Add the aloe vera gel and water to a blender and blend until smooth.
4) Pour the mixture through a strainer or cheesecloth to remove any pulp or solids.
5) Taste the juice and add honey, lemon juice, or other natural sweeteners if desired.
6) Chill the juice in the fridge for at least 30 minutes before serving.

POMEGRANATE JUICE WITH GINGER

Ingredients:

- 2 cups of fresh pomegranate seeds (or 1 cup of pomegranate juice)
- 2 cups of water
- 1-inch piece of fresh ginger root, peeled and chopped
- Honey or other natural sweeteners (optional)

Mixing Guidelines:

1) Rinse the pomegranate seeds and add them to a blender along with the water and chopped ginger.
2) Blend until the mixture is smooth.
3) Pour the mixture through a strainer or cheesecloth to remove any pulp or solids.
4) Taste the juice and add honey or other natural sweeteners if desired.
5) Chill the juice in the fridge for at least 30 minutes before serving.

GREEN JUICE WITH WHEATGRASS AND SPINACH

Ingredients:

- 1 cup of fresh spinach leaves
- 1 ounce of fresh wheatgrass
- 1 green apple, cored and chopped
- 1 cucumber, chopped
- 1 lemon, juiced
- 1-inch piece of fresh ginger root, peeled and chopped
- Water

Mixing Guidelines:

1) Rinse the spinach leaves and wheatgrass.
2) Add the spinach, wheatgrass, apple, cucumber, lemon juice, and ginger to a blender.
3) Add enough water to cover the ingredients.
4) Blend until the mixture is smooth.
5) Pour the mixture through a strainer or cheesecloth to

remove any pulp or solids.

6) Chill the juice in the fridge for at least 30 minutes before serving.

APPLE CIDER VINEGAR AND HONEY DRINK

Ingredients:

- 1 tablespoon of raw, unfiltered apple cider vinegar
- 1 tablespoon of honey
- 1 cup of warm water

Mixing Guidelines:

1) Add the apple cider vinegar and honey to a cup.
2) Pour in the warm water and stir until the honey is dissolved.
3) Drink the mixture slowly.

GOLDEN MILK WITH CINNAMON AND CARDAMOM

Ingredients:

- 1 cup of unsweetened almond milk
- 1 teaspoon of turmeric powder
- 1/4 teaspoon of ground cinnamon
- 1/4 teaspoon of ground cardamom
- 1 teaspoon of honey (optional)

Mixing Guidelines:

1) Add the almond milk, turmeric powder, cinnamon, and cardamom to a small saucepan.
2) Heat the mixture over medium heat, whisking occasionally, until it is warm and well combined.
3) Remove the pan from the heat and let the mixture cool for a few minutes.
4) Stir in the honey (if using).
5) Pour the mixture into a mug and enjoy.

CARROT AND GINGER JUICE

Ingredients:

- 4 large carrots, chopped
- 1 inch piece of fresh ginger, peeled and chopped
- 1/2 cup of water
- 1 tablespoon of honey (optional)

Mixing Guidelines:

1) Add the chopped carrots and ginger to a blender or juicer.
2) Add the water and blend until smooth.
3) Pour the mixture through a fine mesh strainer to remove any pulp.
4) Stir in the honey (if using).
5) Pour the juice into a glass.

HIBISCUS AND ORANGE ICED TEA

Ingredients:

- 4 cups of water
- 4 hibiscus tea bags
- 1 orange, sliced
- 1 tablespoon of honey (optional)

Mixing Guidelines:

1) Bring the water to a boil in a medium-sized saucepan.
2) Remove the pan from the heat and add the hibiscus tea bags and orange slices.
3) Let the mixture steep for 10-15 minutes, until it is well infused.
4) Remove the tea bags and orange slices and let the mixture cool.
5) Stir in the honey (if using).
6) Pour the tea into a pitcher and refrigerate for at least 1 hour.
7) Serve the tea over ice and garnish with additional orange slices, if desired.

CUCUMBER AND LIME INFUSED WATER

Ingredients:

- 1/2 cucumber, sliced
- 1 lime, sliced
- 8 cups of water
- Ice

Mixing Guidelines:

1) Add the cucumber and lime slices to a large pitcher.
2) Fill the pitcher with 8 cups of water.

3) Stir the mixture to combine.
4) Cover the pitcher and refrigerate for at least 1 hour, or overnight.
5) When ready to serve, fill glasses with ice and pour the infused water over the ice.
6) Garnish each glass with additional cucumber and lime slices, if desired.

CRANBERRY AND ORANGE JUICE

Ingredients:

- 2 cups of fresh or frozen cranberries
- 2 oranges, peeled and segmented
- 4 cups of water
- Honey or stevia to taste (optional)

Mixing Guidelines:

1) In a blender, combine the cranberries, oranges, and water.
2) Blend until the mixture is smooth.
3) Pour the mixture through a fine mesh strainer into a pitcher to remove any pulp or seeds.
4) Add honey or stevia to taste, if desired.
5) Stir the mixture to combine.
6) Cover the pitcher and refrigerate until ready to serve.
7) When ready to serve, fill glasses with ice and pour the cranberry and orange juice over the ice.

WATERMELON AND MINT SMOOTHIE

- 3 cups of chopped seedless watermelon
- 1/2 cup of unsweetened almond milk
- 1/2 cup of ice
- 1 tablespoon of honey or stevia to taste (optional)
- 6-8 fresh mint leaves

Mixing Guidelines:

1) In a blender, combine the watermelon, almond milk, ice, and honey or stevia (if using).
2) Blend until the mixture is smooth and creamy.
3) Add the fresh mint leaves to the blender and pulse a few times until they are chopped into small pieces.
4) Pour the smoothie into glasses and garnish with additional fresh mint leaves, if desired.

GINGER AND LEMON TEA WITH HONEY

Ingredients:

- 1-inch piece of fresh ginger, peeled and sliced
- 1 lemon, sliced
- 4 cups of water
- 1-2 tablespoons of honey, to taste (optional)

Mixing Guidelines:

1) In a saucepan, bring the water, ginger, and lemon to a boil.
2) Reduce the heat to low and let the mixture simmer for about 15 minutes.
3) Remove the pan from the heat and let the mixture

cool for a few minutes.

4) Strain the mixture through a fine mesh strainer into a
   teapot or pitcher.
5) Add honey to taste, if desired.
6) Stir the mixture to combine.
7) Serve the ginger and lemon tea hot in teacups.

SWEET POTATO AND CARROT JUICE WITH GINGER

Ingredients:

- 2 sweet potatoes, peeled and chopped
- 4 large carrots, peeled and chopped
- 1-inch piece of fresh ginger, peeled and chopped
- 2 cups of water

Mixing Guidelines:

1) Add the sweet potatoes, carrots, ginger, and water to a
   blender.
2) Blend the mixture until smooth.
3) Strain the mixture through a fine mesh strainer into a
   glass or pitcher.
4) Serve the sweet potato and carrot juice with ginger
   chilled or over ice.

PINEAPPLE AND GINGER JUICE

Ingredients:

- 1 medium-sized pineapple, peeled and cored
- 1-inch piece of fresh ginger, peeled and chopped
- 2 cups of water

Mixing Guidelines:

1) Add the pineapple, ginger, and water to a blender.
2) Blend the mixture until smooth.
3) Strain the mixture through a fine mesh strainer into a glass or pitcher.
4) Serve the pineapple and ginger juice chilled or over ice.

MANGO AND GINGER ICED TEA

Ingredients:

- 2 ripe mangoes, peeled and diced
- 1-inch piece of fresh ginger, peeled and chopped
- 4 cups of water
- 2 bags of black tea
- Honey or stevia (optional)

Mixing Guidelines:

1) In a saucepan, bring the water and ginger to a boil.
2) Reduce the heat and let it simmer for 5 minutes.
3) Remove from heat and add the tea bags. Let it steep for 5 minutes.
4) Remove the tea bags and let the mixture cool to room temperature.
5) In a blender, puree the diced mango until smooth.
6) Strain the mango puree through a fine mesh strainer

to remove any pulp.
7) Mix the mango puree with the cooled ginger tea.
8) Taste and add honey or stevia if desired.
9) Chill the mango and ginger iced tea in the refrigerator.
10) Serve the iced tea over ice

LEMON AND GINGER TURMERIC TONIC

Ingredients:

- 1 lemon, juiced
- 1-inch piece of fresh ginger, peeled and grated
- 1 tsp turmeric powder
- 4 cups of water
- Honey or stevia (optional)

Mixing Guidelines:

1) In a saucepan, bring the water, ginger, and turmeric powder to a boil.
2) Reduce the heat and let it simmer for 5 minutes.
3) Remove from heat and let it cool for a few minutes.
4) Add the lemon juice to the mixture and stir.
5) Taste and add honey or stevia if desired
6) Strain the mixture through a fine mesh strainer.
7) Chill the lemon and ginger turmeric tonic in the refrigerator.
8) Serve the tonic over ice

CINNAMON AND HONEY HOT COCOA

- 2 cups of milk (dairy or non-dairy)
- 2 tbsp unsweetened cocoa powder
- 1/2 tsp ground cinnamon
- 1-2 tbsp honey (adjust to taste)
- Pinch of salt

Mixing Guidelines:

1) In a saucepan, heat the milk over medium heat.
2) Whisk in the cocoa powder, cinnamon, honey, and salt.
3) Continue to whisk the mixture until the cocoa powder has dissolved and the mixture is smooth.
4) Heat the mixture until it's just below boiling, stirring constantly.
5) Pour the hot cocoa into a mug

<h1 style="text-align:center">Chapter 4</h1>

<h2 style="text-align:center">PROBIOTICS FOR STOMACH ULCERS</h2>

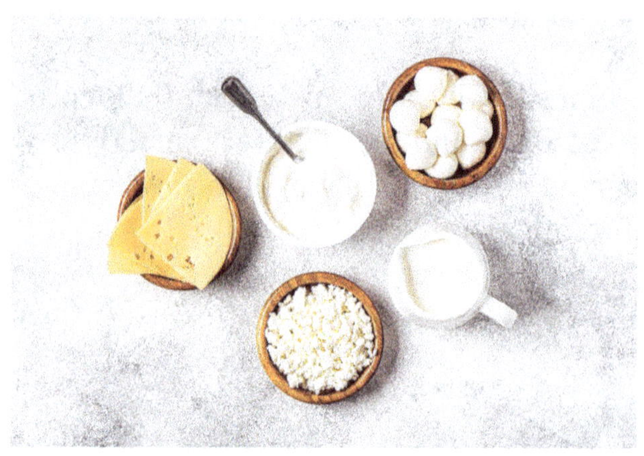

YOGURT PARFAIT

Ingredients:

- 1 cup plain Greek yogurt
- 1/2 cup fresh berries (such as strawberries, blueberries, or raspberries)
- 1/4 cup chopped nuts (such as almonds or walnuts)

- 1-2 tbsp honey (optional)
- Pinch of cinnamon (optional)

Mixing Guidelines:

1) In a small bowl, mix together the Greek yogurt and honey (if using) until well combined.
2) Layer the yogurt mixture, berries, and chopped nuts in a glass or jar.
3) Repeat the layering process until you've used up all the ingredients.
4) Sprinkle a pinch of cinnamon on top if desired.
5) Serve

KEFIR SMOOTHIE

Ingredients:

- 1 cup plain kefir
- 1/2 cup frozen berries (such as blueberries, raspberries, or strawberries)
- 1/2 banana, sliced
- 1 tbsp chia seeds
- 1 tbsp honey (optional)
- 1/4 tsp vanilla extract

Mixing Guidelines:

1) Combine all ingredients in a blender.
2) Blend until smooth and well combined.
3) Pour into a glass

KEFIR SMOOTHIE WITH MANGO AND GINGER

- 1 cup kefir
- 1 cup chopped mango
- 1 tsp grated ginger
- 1 tbsp honey (optional)
- 1/2 cup ice

Mixing Guidelines:

1) In a blender, combine the kefir, chopped mango, grated ginger, and honey (if using).
2) Add the ice and blend until smooth and creamy.
3) Taste and adjust sweetness with more honey if desired.
4) Pour into a glass

BEET AND APPLE KEFIR JUICE

Ingredients:

- 1 medium-sized beet, peeled and chopped
- 1 medium-sized apple, chopped
- 1 cup kefir
- 1 tbsp honey (optional)
- 1/2 cup water
- Juice of 1/2 lemon
- 1/2 tsp grated ginger
- Pinch of salt

1) In a blender, combine the chopped beet, chopped apple, kefir, honey (if using), water, lemon juice, grated ginger, and a pinch of salt.
2) Blend until smooth and creamy.
3) Taste and adjust sweetness with more honey if desired.
4) Pour into a glass

COCONUT WATER KEFIR WITH LEMON

Ingredients:

- 1 cup coconut water
- 1/4 cup water kefir grains
- Juice of 1 lemon
- 1 tsp grated lemon zest
- Optional: honey or maple syrup to sweeten

Mixing Guidelines:

1) In a glass jar, combine the coconut water, water kefir grains, lemon juice, and lemon zest.
2) Cover the jar with a breathable cloth and secure it with a rubber band.
3) Allow the mixture to ferment at room temperature for 24-48 hours, depending on desired taste and fermentation strength.
4) Once the kefir has reached the desired level of tanginess, remove the grains using a non-metal strainer
5) If desired, sweeten with honey or maple syrup to

taste.

6) Transfer the kefir to a bottle or jar with a lid and store
   in the refrigerator until ready to enjoy.
7) Serve chilled

KOMBUCHA WITH GINGER AND TURMERIC

Ingredients:

- 1 SCOBY (Symbiotic Culture Of Bacteria and Yeast)
- 1 cup of sugar
- 8 bags of black tea
- 12 cups of water
- 1 inch of fresh ginger, peeled and grated
- 1 tablespoon of fresh turmeric, grated
- 1/2 cup of Kombucha from a previous batch

Mixing Guidelines:

1) Boil 12 cups of water in a pot, and add 8 bags of black
   tea. Let steep for 5 minutes.
2) Remove the tea bags and stir in 1 cup of sugar until
   dissolved.
3) Allow the tea to cool to room temperature, then
   transfer it to a large glass jar.
4) Add the SCOBY and 1/2 cup of Kombucha from a
   previous batch to the jar.
5) Stir in the grated ginger and turmeric.
6) Cover the jar with a cheesecloth or breathable cloth,
   and secure it with a rubber band.
7) Leave the jar in a warm, dark place for 7-10 days to
   ferment, depending on your taste preference.
8) After the fermentation process is complete, strain the

Kombucha through a fine-mesh strainer to remove any solids.

9) Transfer the Kombucha to bottles or airtight jars and refrigerate until ready to drink.

APPLE CIDER VINEGAR AND HONEY TONIC

Ingredients:

- 2 tablespoons apple cider vinegar
- 1 tablespoon honey
- 1/4 teaspoon ground ginger
- 1/4 teaspoon ground turmeric
- 1/4 teaspoon ground cinnamon
- 1 cup warm water

Mixing Guidelines:

1) In a mug or glass, mix together the apple cider vinegar and honey until the honey has dissolved.
2) Add the ground ginger, turmeric, and cinnamon and stir to combine.
3) Pour in the warm water and stir until everything is well mixed.

TURMERIC AND COCONUT MILK KEFIR

Ingredients:

- 1 cup coconut milk kefir
- 1/2 teaspoon ground turmeric

- 1/4 teaspoon ground cinnamon
- 1 tablespoon honey (optional)

Mixing Guidelines:

1) In a bowl, whisk together the coconut milk kefir, ground turmeric, and ground cinnamon until well combined.
2) If desired, add honey and whisk until fully incorporated.
3) Pour the mixture into a glass

BLUEBERRY KEFIR SMOOTHIE

Ingredients:

- 1 cup blueberries (fresh or frozen)
- 1/2 cup plain kefir
- 1/2 cup almond milk (or other milk of your choice)
- 1 banana
- 1 tablespoon honey (optional)
- 1/2 teaspoon vanilla extract

Mixing Guidelines:

1) Add all the ingredients to a blender and blend until smooth.
2) Taste and adjust sweetness by adding honey if needed.
3) Serve

KEFIR WATER WITH MINT AND CUCUMBER

- 1/2 cup kefir grains
- 1/2 cucumber, sliced
- 1/4 cup fresh mint leaves
- 1/2 cup white sugar
- 1/2 lemon, juiced
- 8 cups filtered water

Mixing Guidelines:

1) In a large glass jar, dissolve the sugar in 4 cups of warm filtered water.
2) Add the remaining 4 cups of cold filtered water and stir to combine.
3) Add the kefir grains to the water and cover the jar with a cheesecloth or coffee filter, secured with a rubber band.
4) Let the mixture ferment at room temperature for 24-48 hours, depending on your taste preference.
5) Once the kefir water has fermented to your liking, strain out the kefir grains and reserve them for the next batch.
6) Add the sliced cucumber, mint leaves, and lemon juice to the kefir water and stir to combine.
7) Serve the kefir water chilled and enjoy the refreshing taste of mint and cucumber.

RASPBERRY KOMBUCHA

Ingredients:

- 1 gallon filtered water
- 1 cup sugar
- 4 black tea bags
- 2 green tea bags
- 1 SCOBY (Symbiotic Culture of Bacteria and Yeast)
- 1 cup pre-made kombucha (as a starter)
- 1 cup raspberries

Mixing Guidelines:

1) Boil 4 cups of water in a pot and steep the black and green tea bags for 5-10 minutes.
2) Remove the tea bags and stir in the sugar until dissolved.
3) Add the remaining gallon of filtered water to the pot and let it cool to room temperature.
4) Once cooled, pour the tea into a large glass jar.
5) Add the SCOBY and pre-made kombucha to the jar, cover it with a cloth, and secure it with a rubber band.
6) Place the jar in a cool, dark place and let it ferment for 7-10 days.
7) After 7-10 days, add the raspberries to the jar.
8) Recover the jar with the cloth and rubber band and let it ferment for another 2-3 days.
9) After the second fermentation, strain the kombucha and raspberries through a fine-mesh strainer and into bottles.
10) Store the bottles in the refrigerator to chill

PINEAPPLE AND GINGER KEFIR

Ingredients:

- 1 cup fresh pineapple chunks
- 1 tsp fresh ginger, grated
- 1 cup milk kefir
- 1 tsp honey (optional)

Mixing Guidelines:

1) In a blender, blend the pineapple chunks and ginger until smooth.
2) In a glass, mix the blended pineapple and ginger with the milk kefir.
3) If desired, add honey to sweeten.

PROBIOTIC ORANGE JUICE WITH FLAXSEED

Ingredients:

- 2 oranges, peeled and segmented
- 1 tablespoon ground flaxseed
- 1 cup plain kefir or kombucha

Mixing Guidelines:

1) In a blender, combine the peeled and segmented oranges and ground flaxseed. Blend until smooth.
2) Pour the orange and flaxseed mixture into a glass.
3) Add the kefir or kombucha to the glass and stir well.
4) Let the mixture sit for a few minutes to allow the flavors to meld together.

5) Drink immediately

FERMENTED CARROT AND GINGER JUICE

- 2 cups of fresh carrot juice
- 1-inch piece of fresh ginger root, peeled and grated
- 1/4 cup of whey or a starter culture
- Pinch of sea salt
- Filtered water

Mixing Guidelines:

1) Combine the fresh carrot juice and grated ginger root in a large glass jar.
2) Add a pinch of sea salt and enough filtered water to fill the jar.
3) Mix in the whey or starter culture and stir well.
4) Cover the jar with a breathable cloth or coffee filter and secure with a rubber band.
5) Let the mixture sit at room temperature for 2-3 days, or until it becomes fizzy and slightly sour.
6) Once the juice is fermented to your liking, transfer it to the refrigerator to slow down the fermentation process.
7) Serve chilled

MANGO AND PINEAPPLE WATER KEFIR

Ingredients:

- 1/4 cup water kefir grains
- 4 cups filtered water
- 1/2 cup chopped pineapple
- 1/2 cup chopped mango
- 1/4 cup organic sugar

Mixing Guidelines:

1) In a clean glass jar, dissolve sugar in filtered water.
2) Add water kefir grains to the jar and cover with a cloth or paper towel, securing it with a rubber band.
3) Allow the mixture to ferment for 24-48 hours at room temperature.
4) After 24-48 hours, remove the kefir grains from the jar using a plastic or wooden spoon and transfer them to a new jar.
5) Add the chopped pineapple and mango to the original jar and cover it with a cloth or paper towel.
6) Allow the fruit mixture to ferment for another 24-48 hours at room temperature.
7) Strain the fruit mixture using a fine mesh strainer and transfer the liquid to a clean jar.
8) Store the mango and pineapple water kefir in the refrigerator

HOMEMADE GINGER BEER

Ingredients:

- 2 cups grated fresh ginger root
- 2 cups sugar
- 1/2 cup fresh lime juice

- 10 cups water
- 1/4 teaspoon active dry yeast

Mixing Guidelines:

1) In a large pot, bring 10 cups of water to a boil.
2) Add 2 cups of grated ginger root and 2 cups of sugar to the pot and stir until the sugar has dissolved.
3) Remove the pot from the heat and let it cool to room temperature.
4) Add 1/4 teaspoon of active dry yeast to the pot and stir.
5) Pour the mixture into a large glass jar and cover the jar with a cloth or cheesecloth.
6) Let the mixture ferment for 2-3 days, stirring it once a day.
7) After 2-3 days, strain the mixture through a fine-mesh strainer and discard the ginger root.
8) Add 1/2 cup of fresh lime juice to the ginger beer and stir.
9) Pour the ginger beer into bottles and store them in the refrigerator.
10) Serve chilled

WATER KEFIR WITH BERRIES AND LEMON

Ingredients:

- ¼ cup water kefir grains
- 4 cups filtered water
- 1 lemon, sliced
- ½ cup mixed berries (strawberries, blueberries, raspberries)

- ¼ cup organic cane sugar
- 1 tablespoon molasses (optional)

1) In a glass jar, dissolve the sugar and molasses in 1 cup of the filtered water. Stir until the sugar is completely dissolved.
2) Add the remaining water to the jar and stir.
3) Add the water kefir grains to the jar and stir gently.
4) Add the sliced lemon and mixed berries to the jar.
5) Cover the jar with a cloth or a lid with an air vent to allow for fermentation.
6) Place the jar in a warm and dark place and let it ferment for 24-48 hours.
7) After 24-48 hours, strain the water kefir using a fine-mesh strainer.
8) Transfer the strained water kefir to a clean jar and store it in the refrigerator.

CUCUMBER AND MINT KOMBUCHA

Ingredients:

- 1 cup kombucha
- 1 cup water
- 1/2 cup sliced cucumber
- 4-5 mint leaves
- 1 tbsp honey (optional)

Mixing Guidelines:

1) In a blender, blend together the cucumber and mint

leaves with a little bit of water until smooth.

2) In a glass jar or bottle, combine the blended cucumber and mint mixture, kombucha, and water.

3) If desired, add honey and stir until dissolved.

4) Cover the jar or bottle with a cheesecloth or coffee filter and secure with a rubber band.

5) Leave the mixture to ferment at room temperature for 1-3 days.

6) After fermentation, remove the cheesecloth or coffee filter and replace with a lid.

7) Store the kombucha in the fridge for up to a week.

8) Serve chilled

FERMENTED SWEET POTATO JUICE WITH CINNAMON

Ingredients:

- 2-3 sweet potatoes
- 1 cinnamon stick
- 1-2 cups of filtered water
- 1/4 cup of coconut sugar (optional)

Mixing Guidelines:

1) Wash the sweet potatoes and cut them into small pieces.

2) Put the sweet potatoes and cinnamon stick into a large glass jar.

3) Add filtered water until the jar is almost full.

4) If you want to add some sweetness to your drink, add coconut sugar to the mixture.

5) Stir the mixture well to dissolve the sugar.

6) Cover the jar with a cheesecloth or a paper towel and secure it with a rubber band.

7) Leave the mixture at room temperature for 2-3 days to ferment.

8) After 2-3 days, strain the mixture through a fine mesh strainer or cheesecloth.

9) Pour the fermented sweet potato juice into a glass bottle and store it in the fridge.

PROBIOTIC HOT CHOCOLATE WITH CINNAMON

Ingredients:

- 2 cups milk (dairy or non-dairy)
- 2 tbsp unsweetened cocoa powder
- 1-2 tbsp maple syrup or honey (to taste)
- 1 tsp vanilla extract
- 1/2 tsp ground cinnamon
- 1/2 cup kefir or plain yogurt

Mixing Guidelines:

1) In a small saucepan, whisk together milk, cocoa powder, maple syrup or honey, vanilla extract, and ground cinnamon.

2) Heat the mixture over medium-low heat, whisking constantly until it is hot and steamy, but not boiling.

3) Remove the pan from the heat and let it cool slightly.

4) Once the mixture has cooled down a bit, whisk in the kefir or yogurt.

5) Pour the hot chocolate into two mugs and serve right away.

PROBIOTIC LEMONADE WITH HONEY AND GINGER

Ingredients:

- 1 cup fresh lemon juice
- 4 cups filtered water
- 1/4 cup raw honey
- 1/2 cup ginger bug (or 1/4 cup whey or 1/4 cup kombucha)
- Ice cubes
- Sliced lemons and ginger, for garnish (optional)

Mixing Guidelines:

1) In a large pitcher, mix together the lemon juice, filtered water, and raw honey until well combined.
2) Add in the ginger bug and stir well.
3) Refrigerate the lemonade for 1-2 days, allowing it to ferment and develop a slight fizziness. Note: If using whey or kombucha, the fermentation time may vary.
4) Once the lemonade is fermented to your liking, give it a stir and pour over ice cubes.
5) Garnish with sliced lemons and ginger, if desired.

Final Thoughts and Recommendations

Congrats on completing your transition to a healthy lifestyle! It might be difficult but worthwhile to include smoothies and other beverages that are good for stomach ulcers in your regular diet. Just keep in mind that the improvements you make now will benefit your health for years to come.

If you mess up or have a poor day, don't give up. Keep in mind that the goal is growth, not perfection. It involves implementing minor adjustments each day and maintaining them over time. Key is consistency.

Do not forget to pay attention to your body and modify your food as necessary. Since every individual has a unique nature, what works for one person may not work for another. Try out several smoothies and beverages to see which suits you the best.

Adding a variety of fruits, vegetables, and herbs into your

diet not only aids in the treatment of stomach ulcers, but also delivers critical nutrients that promote general health and well-being. So continue experimenting with new dishes and tastes.

Last but not least, remember to have fun on the way! Accept the different tastes and sensations that a healthy diet brings. Appreciate your accomplishments and keep in mind that even the smallest steps may lead to a healthier you.

Cheers to your wellbeing and health!

ABOUT THE AUTHOR

Aashvi Dhingra is an India born woman who currently resides in the United States. Aashvi has always been passionate about food and nutrition, which led her to pursue a career as a Registered Dietitian. Aashvi earned her Bachelor's degree in Nutrition and Dietetics from a prestigious university in India, and later received her Master's degree in Nutrition Science from a renowned university in the United States.

Aashvi's journey as a dietitian began in India, where she worked in various clinical and community settings. During her time in India, Aashvi developed a keen interest in the intersection between food, culture, and health. She conducted several research studies on the impact of traditional Indian diets on health outcomes, which earned her recognition and awards from various academic and research organizations.

In the United States, Aashvi has worked as a clinical dietitian in a hospital setting, where she has helped patients with various health conditions achieve their nutrition goals. Aashvi has also worked with several community organizations to promote healthy eating habits and improve access to nutritious foods.

Apart from her professional work as a dietitian, Aashvi is an avid home cook who loves experimenting with new recipes and flavors. She believes that cooking is a creative and therapeutic process that brings people together and fosters cultural exchange. Aashvi often shares her recipes and cooking tips on her social media platforms and has gained a significant following.

Aashvi's multicultural background and experience as a dietitian have shaped her approach to food and nutrition. She believes that a healthy and balanced diet should be personalized to an individual's cultural background, preferences, and lifestyle. Aashvi also emphasizes the importance of food education and empowering individuals to make informed choices about their diet.

Through her work as a dietitian and her passion for cooking, Aashvi hopes to inspire others to prioritize their health and well-being through food. She also aims to promote cultural understanding and celebrate the diversity of cuisines and culinary traditions around the world.

In her free time, Aashvi enjoys traveling, hiking, and exploring new restaurants and food markets. She is also an avid reader and enjoys learning about new topics related to food, culture, and health.